Air Fryer Budget Friendly Cookbook

Over 50 New And Delicious Recipes For Your Air Fryer

Joana Smith

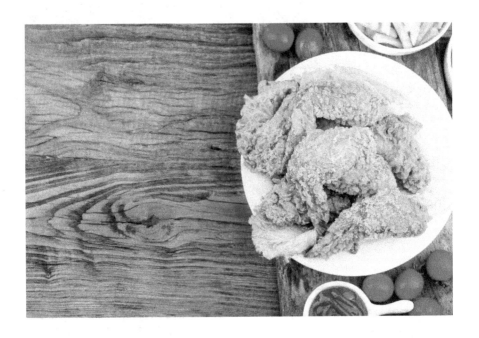

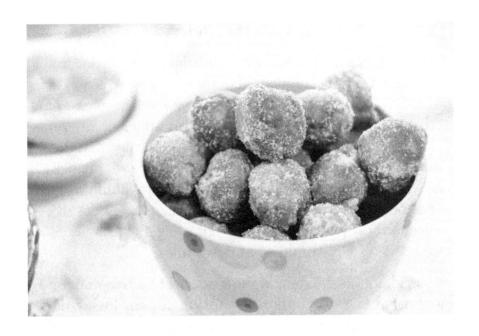

Table Of Contents

DESCRIPTION 8

INTRODUCTION 10

CHAPTER 1 BREAKFAST 12

   1.   BLACK BEAN CHEESE BURRITOS 12

   2.   MUSHROOM TOFU CASSEROLE 14

   3.   ALSA OMELET 17

CHAPTER 2 MAINS 18

   4.   CEDAR PLANKED SALMON 18

   5.   CRESTED HALIBUT 20

   6.   CREAMY HALIBUT 22

   7.   EGGPLANT FRIES 23

   8.   AIR FRIED PITA BREAD PIZZA 24

   9.   LIGHT & CRISPY OKRA 25

CHAPTER 3 SIDES 28

   10.   CRISPY BLACK-EYED PEAS 28

   11.   SPICY MOZZARELLA STICK 30

CHAPTER 4 SEAFOOD 32

   12.   GINGER SALMON MIX 32

   13.   SALMON FILLETS AND GREEN OLIVES 34

   14.   CHERVIL COD 35

CHAPTER 5 POULTRY 36

15. HONEY-BALSAMIC ORANGE CHICKEN 36

16. SALSA VERDE OVER GRILLED CHICKEN 38

17. CHICKEN GRILL RECIPE FROM CALIFORNIA 40

18. TURKEY CHILI 42

CHAPTER 6 MEAT 44

19. LAMB WITH PEAS AND TOMATOES 44

20. LAMB WITH ZUCCHINIS AND EGGPLANTS MIX 46

21. BEEF WITH BEANS 48

22. GREEK BEEF MIX 50

23. BEEF AND FENNEL 51

24. LAMB AND EGGPLANT MEATLOAF 53

CHAPTER 7 VEGETABLES 56

25. SAVOY CABBAGE 56

26. AVOCADO FRIES 58

27. CRISPY FRENCH FRIES 60

CHAPTER 8 SNACKS 62

28. SEA SALT AND BLACK PEPPER CUCUMBER CHIPS 62

29. EASY BUTTERED-MUSHROOM CAKES 64

30. DELICIOUS BEET WEDGES DISH 66

31. CHILI LIME BROCCOLI CRUNCH 67

32. ZUCCHINI CHIPS 69

33. CRUSTLESS PIZZA 71

34. OLIVES AND ZUCCHINI CAKES 73

35. TOMATO BITES 75

36. SPINACH ROLLS 77

37. RANCH ROASTED ALMONDS 79

CHAPTER 9 DESSERT 80

38. CASHEW DIP 80

39. SMOKED SALMON SALAD 82

40. SALMON MEATBALLS 84

41. CHICKEN MEATBALLS 86

42. GINGER DIP 88

43. ASPARAGUS AND OLIVES BOWLS 90

44. WALNUTS AND RADISH BITES 92

45. BREAD PUDDING 93

46. ALMOND AND COCOA CAKE 95

47. BLUEBERRY CAKE 97

48. PEACH CINNAMON COBBLER 99

49. EASY PEARS DESSERT 101

50. STRAWBERRY CHEESECAKE 102

51. CHERRIES AND RHUBARB BOWLS 104

52. CHOCOLATE CHIPS CREAM 105

DAY MEAL PLAN 106

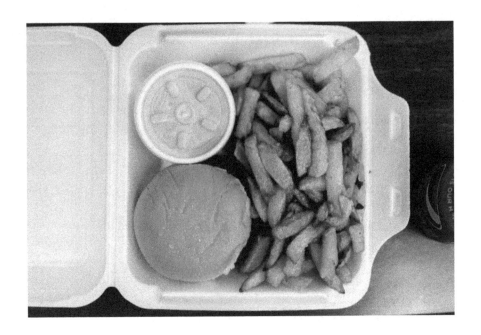

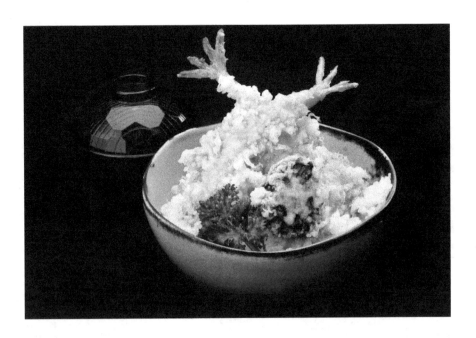

DESCRIPTION

The history of Air fryers dates back to a few years ago; exactly during the third quarter of the year 2010 and it was a completely revolutionary invention that was invented by Philips Electronics Company. Philips introduced the Air Fryer to the world and changed the conception of the culinary world all at once.

The Air Fryer is used as a substitute for your oven, stovetop, and deep fryer. It comes with various handy parts and other tools that you can buy to use your Air Fryer for different cooking styles, which include the following:

• Grilling. It provides the same heat to grill food ingredients without the need to flip them continuously. The hot air goes around the fryer, giving heating on all sides. The recipes include directions of how many times you ought to shake the pan during the cooking process.
To make the process of grilling faster, you can use a grill pan or a grill layer. They will soak the excess fat from the meat that you are cooking to give you delicious and healthy meals.

• Baking. The Air Fryer usually comes with a baking pan (or you can buy or use your own to make treats that are typically done using an oven. You can bake goodies, such as cakes, bread, cupcakes, muffins, and brownies in your Air Fryer.
• Roasting. It roasts food ingredients, which include vegetables and meat, faster than when you do it in the oven.
• Frying is its primary purpose – to cook fried foods with little or no oil.
You can cook most food items in an Air Fryer. There are some foods that you should refrain from cooking in the fryer because they will taste better when cooked in the traditional ways — they include fried foods with batter and steamed veggies, such as beans and carrots.

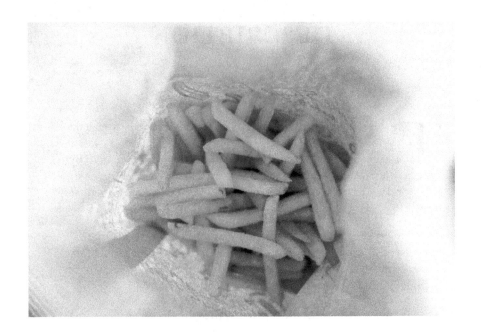

INTRODUCTION

There are many kinds of foods that you can cook using an air fryer, but there are also certain types that are not suited for it. Avoid cooking ingredients, which can be steamed, like beans and carrots. You also cannot fry foods covered in heavy batter in this appliance.

Aside from the above mentioned, you can cook most kinds of ingredients using an air fryer. You can use it to cook foods covered in light flour or breadcrumbs. You can cook a variety of vegetables in the appliance, such as cauliflower, asparagus, zucchini, kale, peppers, and corn on the cob. You can also use it to cook frozen foods and home prepared meals by following a different set of instructions for these purposes.

An air fryer also comes with another useful feature - the separator. It allows you to cook multiple dishes at a time. Use the separator to divide ingredients in the pan or basket. You have to make sure that all ingredients have the same temperature setting so that everything will cook evenly at the same time.

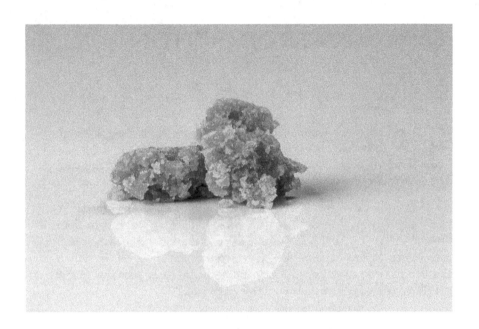

CHAPTER 1

BREAKFAST

1. Black Bean Cheese Burritos

Preparation Time: 19 Minutes • Servings: 2

INGREDIENTS

- Canned black beans, drained-2 cups

- Olive oil- a drizzle

- Red bell pepper, sliced -½

- Small avocado, peeled, pitted and sliced- 1

- Mild salsa -2 tbsp.

- Salt and black pepper- to taste

- Mozzarella cheese, shredded-⅛ cup

- Tortillas -2

DIRECTIONS

1. Grease your Air fryer pan with oil.

2. Add beans, salsa, salt, pepper, and bell peppers.

3. Seal the fryer and cook for 6minutes at 400 o F on Air fryer mode.

4. Spread the tortillas on the working surface then divide the beans mixture on top.

5. Add avocado and cheese, then roll the burritos.

6. Place the burritos in the Air fryer basket and seal the fryer.

7. Cook for 3 minutes at 300 o F on Air fryer mode.

8. Serve.

NUTRITION: Calories: 189, Fat: 3g, Fiber: 7g, Carbs: 12g, Protein: 5g

2. Mushroom Tofu Casserole

Preparation Time: 35 Minutes • Servings: 2

INGREDIENTS

- Yellow onion, chopped -1

- Garlic, minced-1 tbsp.

- Olive oil-1 tbsp.

- Carrot, chopped -1

- Celery stalks, chopped-2

- White mushrooms, chopped-½ cup

- Red bell pepper, chopped -½ cup

- Salt and black pepper- to taste

- Oregano, a dried-1 tbsp.

- Cumin, a ground-½ tbsp.

- Firm tofu, cubed-7 ounces

- Lemon juice -1 tbsp.

- Water -2 tbsp.

- Quinoa, already cooked-½ cup

- Cheddar cheese, grated-2 tbsp.

DIRECTIONS

1. Choose a pan and grease it with oil. Place it over medium heat.

2. Add onion and garlic. Sauté for 3 minutes.

3. Stir in celery, carrots, bell peppers, salt, mushrooms, pepper, cumin, and oregano.

4. Sauté for 6 minutes then take it off the heat.

5. Add tofu to the food processor along with cheese, quinoa, water, and lemon juice.

6. Blend until it is smooth then add this mixture to the sautéed veggies.

7. Mix well then add these veggies to the Air fryer pan.

8. Seal the Air fryer and cook for 15 minutes at 350 o F on Air fryer mode.

9. Serve warm.

NUTRITION: Calories: 230, Fat: 11g, Fiber: 7g, Carbs: 14g, Protein: 5g

3. Alsa Omelet

Preparation time: 5 minutes • Cooking time: 20 minutes

• Servings:

INGREDIENTS

- 8 eggs, whisked 1 cup mild salsa

- 4 scallions, chopped 1 tablespoon parsley, chopped Cooking spray

- ¼ cup mozzarella, shredded

- Salt and black pepper to the taste

DIRECTIONS

1. Heat up the air fryer at 360 degrees F, grease it with the cooking spray, add the eggs mixed with the salsa and the other ingredients, spread, cook for 20 minutes, divide between plates and serve.

NUTRITION: Calories 230, Fat 14, Fiber 3, Carbs 5, Protein 11

CHAPTER 2

MAINS

4. Cedar Planked Salmon

Cooking Time: 15 minutes • Servings: 6

INGREDIENTS

- 4 untreated cedar planks

- ½ cup olive oil

- 1½ tablespoons of rice vinegar

- 1 teaspoon sesame oil

- 2 lbs. of salmon fillets, skin removed

- 1 teaspoon garlic, minced

- 1 tablespoon ginger root, fresh, grated

- ¼ cup green onions, chopped

- ½ cup soy sauce

DIRECTIONS

1. Start by soaking the cedar planks for 2- hours. Take a shallow baking dish and stir in the olive oil, the rice vinegar, the sesame oil, soy sauce, ginger, and green onions. Place the salmon fillets in the prepared marinade for at least 20- minutes. Place the planks in the basket of your air fryer. Cook the salmon fillets for 15-minutes at 360°Fahrenheit.

NUTRITION: Calories: 273, Total Fat: 7.5g, Carbs: 5.2g, Protein: 34.2g

5. Crested Halibut

Cooking Time: 30 minutes Servings: 4

INGREDIENTS

- 4halibut fillets

- ¾ cup of pork rinds

- ½ cup of parsley, fresh, chopped

- ¼ cup dill, fresh, chopped

- ¼ cup chives, fresh, chopped

- 1tablespoon olive oil

- 1teaspoon lemon zest, finely grated

- Sea salt and black pepper to taste

DIRECTIONS

1. Preheat your air fryer to 390°Fahrenheit. In a mixing bowl, combine the pork rinds, parsley, dill, chives, olive oil, lemon zest, sea salt and black pepper. Rinse the halibut fillets

and dry them on a paper towel. Arrange the halibut fillets and dry them on a paper towel. Arrange the halibut fillets onto a baking sheet. Spoon the pork rind crumb mixture onto fish fillets. Lightly press the mixture on the fillets. Bake the fillets in your preheated air fryer basket for 30- minutes. Serve warm.

NUTRITION: Calories: 272, Total Fat:10.3g, Carbs: 9.4g, Protein: 32.2g

6. Creamy Halibut

Cooking Time: 20 minutes • Servings: 6

INGREDIENTS

- 2lbs. of halibut fillets, cut into 6 pieces

- 1teaspoon dill weed, dried ½ cup light sour cream ½ cup light mayonnaise

- 4chopped green onions

DIRECTIONS

1. Preheat the air fryer to 390°Fahrenheit. Season the halibut with salt and pepper. In a bowl, mix the onions, sour cream, mayonnaise, and dill. Spread the onion mixture evenly over the halibut fillets. Cook in air fryer for 20-minutes. Serve warm.

NUTRITION: Calories:286, Total Fat: 11.3g, Carbs: 6.9, Protein: 29.8g

7. Eggplant Fries

Cooking Time: 20 minutes • Servings: 4

INGREDIENTS

- 1eggplant, cut into 3-inch pieces

- ¼ cup of water

- 1tablespoon of olive oil

- 4tablespoons cornstarch

- sea salt to taste

DIRECTIONS

1. Preheat your air fryer to 390°Fahrenheit. In a bowl, combine eggplant, water, oil and cornstarch. Place the eggplant fries in air fryer basket, and air fry them for 20- minutes. Serve warm and enjoy!

8. Air Fried Pita Bread Pizza

Cooking Time: 6 minutes • Servings: 3

INGREDIENTS

- 1large pita bread 1teaspoon olive oil

- 7pepperoni slices ¼ cup of sausage

- ½ teaspoon garlic, minced

- 1tablespoon pizza sauce

- ¼ cup mozzarella cheese, shredded

- 1small onion, finely diced

DIRECTIONS

1. Spread the pizza sauce over the pita bread evenly. Arrange pepperoni, onion, and sausage over pita bread. Sprinkle the top with garlic and cheese. Drizzle the pizza with olive oil then place in air basket. Place on top of trivet and air fry at 350°Fahrenheit for 6-minutes. Serve and enjoy!

9. Light & Crispy Okra

Cooking Time: 10 minutes Servings: 4

INGREDIENTS

- 3cups okra, wash and dry

- 1teaspoon fresh lemon juice

- 1teaspoon coriander

- 3tablespoons gram flour

- 2teaspoons red chili powder

- 1teaspoon dry mango powder

- 1teaspoon cumin powder

- Sea salt to taste

DIRECTIONS

1. Cut the top of okra then cut a deep horizontal cut in each okra and set aside. In a bowl, combine gram flour, salt, lemon juice, and all the spices. Add a little water in gram flour mixture and make a thick batter.

Fill batter in each okra and place in the air fryer basket. Spray okra with cooking spray. Preheat your air fryer to 350°Fahrenheit for 5-minutes. Air fry the stuffed okra for 10-minutes or until lightly golden brown. Serve and enjoy!

NUTRITION: Calories: 56, Total Fat: 0.8g, Carbs: 9g, Protein: 2g

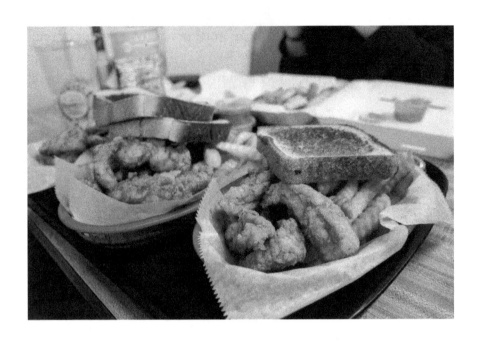

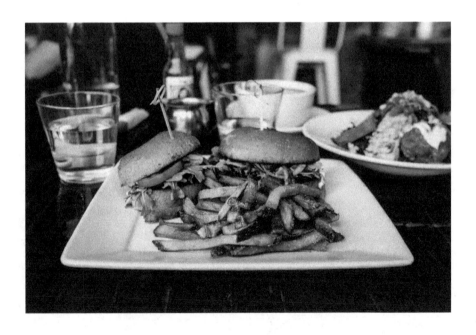

CHAPTER 3

SIDES

10.   Crispy Black-Eyed Peas

Cooking Time: 10 minutes • Servings: 6

INGREDIENTS

- 15-ounces black-eyed peas

- 1/8 teaspoon chipotle chili powder

- ¼ teaspoon salt

- ½ teaspoon chili powder

- 1/8 teaspoon black pepper

DIRECTIONS

1. Rinse the beans well with running water then set

    aside. In a large bowl, mix the spices until well

    combined. Add the peas to spices and mix. Place

the peas in the wire basket and cook for 10-

minutes at 360°Fahrenheit. Serve and enjoy!

NUTRITION: Calories: 262,   Total   Fat:

9.4g, Carbs: 8.6g, Protein: 9.2g

11. Spicy Mozzarella Stick

Cooking Time: 5 minutes • Servings: 3

INGREDIENTS

- 8-ounces mozzarella cheese, cut into strips

- 2tablespoons olive oil

- ½ teaspoon salt

- 1cup pork rinds

- 1egg

- 1teaspoon garlic powder

- 1teaspoon paprika

DIRECTIONS

1. Cut the mozzarella into 6 strips. Whisk the egg along with salt, paprika, and garlic powder. Dip the mozzarella strips into egg mixture first, then into pork rinds. Arrange them on a baking platter and place in the fridge for 30-

minutes. Preheat your air fryer to 360°Fahrenheit. Drizzle olive oil into the air fryer. Arrange the mozzarella sticks in the air fryer and cook for about 5- minutes. Make sure to turn them at least twice, to ensure they will become golden on all sides.

NUTRITION: Calories: 156, Total Fat: 9.6g, Carbs: 1.89g, Protein: 16g

CHAPTER 4

SEAFOOD

12.   Ginger Salmon Mix

Preparation time: 4 minutes • Cooking time: 15 minutes

• Servings: 4

INGREDIENTS

- 1pound salmon fillets, boneless

- 1tablespoon ginger, grated

- 1tablespoon olive oil

- 2teaspoons garlic powder

- 1tablespoon lemon juice

- 1tablespoon dill, chopped

- Salt and black pepper to the taste

DIRECTIONS

1. In the air fryer's pan, mix the salmon with the ginger and the other ingredients, toss, introduce the pan in the air fryer and cook at 380 degrees F for 15 minutes.

2. Divide between plates and serve..

NUTRITION: Calories 236, Fat 8, Fiber 12, Carbs 17, Protein 16

13.   Salmon Fillets and Green Olives

Preparation time: 4 minutes • Cooking time: 20 minutes

• Servings: 4

INGREDIENTS

- 1cup green olives, pitted 1pound salmon fillets, boneless Salt and black pepper to the taste

- 1tablespoon avocado oil Juice of 1 lime

- 1tablespoon dill, chopped

DIRECTIONS

1. In a baking dish that fits your air fryer, mix the salmon with the green olives and the other ingredients, toss gently, introduce in your air fryer and cook at 370 degrees F for 20 minutes.

2. Divide everything between plates and serve.

NUTRITION: Calories 281, Fat 8, Fiber 14, Carbs 17, Protein 16

14. Chervil Cod

Preparation time: 10 minutes • Cooking time: 20 minutes • Servings: 4

INGREDIENTS

- 4cod fillets, boneless 1tablespoon chervil, chopped
- Juice of 1 lime Salt and black pepper to the taste
- ½ cup coconut milk
- A drizzle of olive oil

DIRECTIONS

1. In a baking dish that fits your air fryer, mix the cod with the chervil and the other ingredients, toss gently, introduce in your air fryer and cook at 380 degrees F for 20 minutes.

2. Divide between plates and serve hot.

NUTRITION: Calories 250, Fat 5, Fiber 6, Carbs 15, Protein 18

CHAPTER 5

POULTRY

15.   Honey-Balsamic Orange Chicken

Servings: 3 • Cooking Time: 40 minutes

INGREDIENTS

- ½ cup balsamic vinegar ½ cup honey

- 1½ pounds boneless chicken breasts, pounded

- 1tablespoon orange zest 1teaspoon fresh oregano, chopped 2tablespoons extra virgin olive oil

- Salt and pepper to taste

DIRECTIONS:

1. Put the chicken in a Ziploc bag and pour over the rest of the Ingredients. Shake to combine everything.

Allow to marinate in the fridge for at least 2 hours.

2. Preheat the air fryer to 3900F.

3. Place the grill pan accessory in the air fryer.

4. Grill the chicken for 40 minutes.

NUTRITION: Calories: 521; Carbs: 56.1g; Protein: 51.8g; Fat: 9.9g

16.   Salsa Verde Over Grilled Chicken

Servings: 2 • Cooking Time: 40 minutes

INGREDIENTS

- ½ red onion, chopped
- ½ teaspoon chili powder
- 1 jalapeno thinly sliced
- 1 jar salsa verde, divided
- 1-pound boneless skinless chicken breasts
- 2 cloves of garlic, minced
- 2 tablespoons chopped cilantro
- 2 tablespoons extra virgin olive oil
- 4 slices Monterey Jack cheese
- Juice from ½ lime
- Lime wedges for serving

DIRECTIONS:

1. In a Ziploc bag, add half of the salsa verde,

olive oil, lime juice, garlic, chili powder and chicken. Allow to marinate in the fridge for at least 2 hours.

2   Preheat the air fryer to 3900F.

3   Place the grill pan accessory in the air fryer.

4   Grill the chicken for 40 minutes.

5   Flip the chicken every 10 minutes to cook evenly.

6   Serve the chicken with the cheese, jalapeno, red onion, cilantro, and lime wedges.

NUTRITION: Calories: 541; Carbs: 4.5g; Protein: 65.3g; Fat: 29.1g

17. Chicken Grill Recipe from California

Servings: 4 • Cooking Time: 40 minutes

INGREDIENTS

- ¾ cup balsamic vinegar
- 1teaspoon garlic powder
- 2tablespoons extra virgin olive oil
- 2tablespoons honey
- 2teaspoons Italian seasoning
- 4boneless chicken breasts
- 4slices mozzarella
- 4slices of avocado
- 4slices tomato
- Balsamic vinegar for drizzling
- Salt and pepper to taste

DIRECTIONS:

1. In a Ziploc bag, mix together the balsamic vinegar, garlic powder, honey, olive oil, Italian seasoning, salt, pepper, and chicken.

2. Allow to marinate in the fridge for at least 2 hours.

3. Preheat the air fryer to 3900F.

4. Place the grill pan accessory in the air fryer.

5. Put the chicken on the grill and cook for 40 minutes.

6. Flip the chicken every 10 minutes to grill all sides evenly.

7. Serve the chicken with mozzarella, avocado, and tomato. Drizzle with balsamic vinegar.

NUTRITION: Calories: 853;   Carbs:43.2g; Protein:69.4 g; Fat: 44.7g

18.   Turkey Chili

Preparation time: 10 minutes • Cooking time: 25 minutes • Servings: 4

INGREDIENTS

- 1pound turkey breast, skinless, boneless and cubed
- 1red onion, chopped
- 1red chili pepper, minced
- 1cup tomato sauce
- 1teaspoon chili powder
- Salt and black pepper to the taste
- 1teaspoon cumin, ground
- 1cup chicken stock

DIRECTIONS

1. In a pan that fits your air fryer, mix the turkey with the onion and the other ingredients, stir,

introduce in the fryer and cook at 380 degrees

F for 25 minutes.

2   Divide into bowls and serve.

NUTRITION: Calories 251, Fat 8, Fiber 8, Carbs 15,

Protein 17

CHAPTER 6

MEAT

19.   Lamb with Peas and Tomatoes

Preparation time: 10 minutes • Cooking time: 30 minutes • Servings: 4

INGREDIENTS

- 2pounds lamb stew meat, cubed

- 1cup peas

- 1cup canned tomatoes, crushed

- 1cup spring onions, chopped

- 2tablespoons tomato paste

- 3garlic cloves, minced

- A pinch of salt and black pepper

- ½ teaspoon coriander, ground

DIRECTIONS

1. In a pan that fits your air fryer, mix the lamb with the peas and the other ingredients, toss, introduce in the fryer and cook at 390 degrees F for 30 minutes.

2. Divide everything into bowls and serve.

NUTRITION: Calories 289, Fat 8, Fiber 12, Carbs 20, Protein 19

20. Lamb with Zucchinis and Eggplants Mix

Preparation time: 10 minutes • Cooking time: 30 minutes • Servings: 4

INGREDIENTS

- 1pound lamb stew meat, cubed

- 2zucchinis, cubed

- 2eggplants, cubed

- 4garlic cloves, minced

- 2tablespoons avocado oil

- ½ teaspoon coriander, ground

- 1teaspoon nutmeg, ground

- A pinch of salt and black pepper

- ½ cup beef stock

DIRECTIONS

1. In a pan that fits your air fryer mix the lamb

with the zucchinis, eggplants and the other ingredients, introduce in the fryer and cook at 400 degrees F for 30 minutes, shaking the fryer halfway.

2 Divide everything between plates and serve.

NUTRITION: Calories 293, Fat 12, Fiber 12, Carbs 20, Protein 29

21.   Beef with Beans

Preparation time: 10 minutes Cooking time: 30 minutes

Servings: 4

INGREDIENTS

- 2pounds beef stew meat, cubed

- 1cups canned kidney beans, drained

- 1teaspoon sweet paprika

- ½ teaspoon coriander, ground

- 2tablespoons olive oil

- 1cup tomato sauce

- Salt and black pepper to the taste

- 1tablespoon chives, chopped

DIRECTIONS

1. In baking dish that fits your air fryer, mix the beef
   with the beans and the other ingredients,
   introduce the dish in the fryer and cook at 390

degrees F for 30 minutes

2   ivide everything into bowls and serve.

NUTRITION: Calories 275, Fat 3, Fiber 7, Carbs 20,

Protein 18

22.   **Greek Beef Mix**

Preparation time: 5 minutes • Cooking time: 30 minutes

• Servings: 4 INGREDIENTS:

- 2pounds beef stew meat, roughly cubed

- 1teaspoon coriander, ground

- 1teaspoon garam masala 1teaspoon cumin, ground

- A pinch of salt and black pepper

- 1cup Greek yogurt

- ½ teaspoon turmeric powder

DIRECTIONS

1. In the air fryer's pan, mix the beef with the coriander and the other ingredients, toss and cook at 380 degrees F for 30 minutes.

2. Divide between plates and serve.

NUTRITION: Calories 283, Fat 13, Fiber 3, Carbs 6, Protein 15

23. Beef and Fennel

Preparation time: 5 minutes • Cooking time: 30 minutes

• Servings: 4

INGREDIENTS

- 2pounds beef stew meat, cut into strips

- 2fennel bulbs, sliced

- 2tablespoons mustard

- A pinch of salt and black pepper

- 1tablespoon black peppercorns, ground

- 2tablespoons balsamic vinegar

- 2tablespoons olive oil

DIRECTIONS

1. In the air fryer's pan, mix the beef with the fennel and the other ingredients.

2. Put the pan in the fryer and cook at 380 degrees for 30 minutes.

3. Divide everything into bowls and serve.

NUTRITION: Calories 283, Fat 13, Fiber 2, Carbs 6, Protein 17

24.   Lamb and Eggplant Meatloaf

Preparation time: 5 minutes • Cooking time: 35 minutes

• Servings: 4

INGREDIENTS

- 2pounds lamb stew meat, ground

- 2eggplants, chopped

- 1yellow onion, chopped

- A pinch of salt and black pepper

- ½ teaspoon coriander, ground

- Cooking spray

- 2tablespoons cilantro, chopped

- 1egg

- 2tablespoons tomato paste

DIRECTIONS

1. In a bowl, mix the lamb with the eggplants of the ingredients except the cooking spray and

stir.

2. Grease a loaf pan that fits the air fryer with the cooking spray, add the mix and shape the meatloaf.

3. Put the pan in the air fryer and cook at 380 degrees F for 35 minutes.

4. Slice and serve with a side salad.

NUTRITION: Calories 263, Fat 12, Fiber 3, Carbs 6, Protein 15

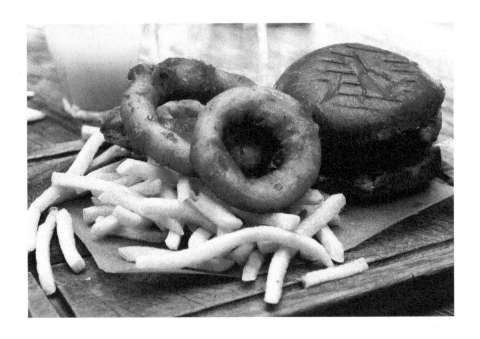

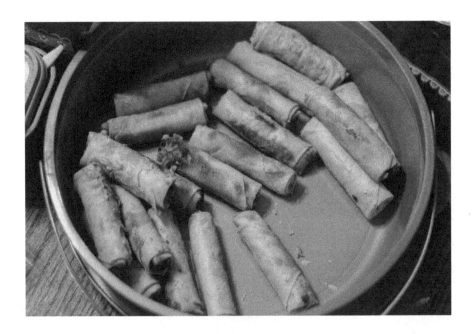

CHAPTER 7

VEGETABLES

25.   Savoy Cabbage

Preparation Time: 20 minutes • Servings: 4

INGREDIENTS

- 1Savoy cabbage head, shredded

- 1tbsp. dill; chopped.

- 1½ tbsp. ghee; melted

- ¼ cup coconut cream

- Salt and black pepper to taste.

DIRECTIONS

1. In a pan that fits the air fryer, combine all the ingredients except the coconut cream, toss, put the pan in the air fryer and cook at 390°F for 10 minutes

2 Add the cream, toss, cook for 5 minutes more, divide between plates and serve

NUTRITION: Calories: 173; Fat: 5g; Fiber: 3g; Carbs: 5g; Protein: 8g

26.   Avocado Fries

Preparation time: 5 minutes • Cooking time: 10 minutes

• Servings: 1

INGREDIENTS:

- 1egg

- 1ripe avocado

- ½ tsp salt

- ½ cup of panko breadcrumbs

DIRECTION:

1. Preheat the air fryer to 400°F (200°Cfor 5 minutes.

2. Remove the avocado pit and cut into fries. In a small bowl, whisk the egg with the salt.

3. Enter the breadcrumbs on a plate.

4. Dip the quarters in the egg mixture, then in the breadcrumbs.

5. Put them in the fryer. Cook for 8-10 minutes.

6. Turn halfway through cooking.

NUTRITION: Calories 390 Fat 32g Carbohydrates 24g

Sugars 3g Protein 4g Cholesterol 0mg

27. Crispy French Fries

Preparation time: 5 minutes • Cooking time: 10 minutes

• Servings: 2

INGREDIENTS

- 2medium sweet potatoes

- 2tsp olive oil

- ½ tsp salt

- ½ tsp garlic powder

- ¼ tsp paprika

- Black pepper

DIRECTION:

1. Preheat the hot air fryer to 400°F (200°C

2. Spray the basket with a little oil.

3. Cut the sweet potatoes into potato chips about 1 cm wide.

4. Add oil, salt, garlic powder, pepper and

paprika.

5. Cook for 8 minutes, without overloading the basket.

6. Repeat 2 or 3 times, as necessary.

NUTRITION: Calories 240 Fat 9g Carbohydrates 36g Sugars 1g Protein 3g Cholesterol 0mg

CHAPTER 8

SNACKS

28. Sea Salt and Black Pepper Cucumber Chips

Preparation time: 15 minutes • Cooking time: 3 Hours • Servings: 4

INGREDIENTS

- 4cups very thin cucumber slices

- 2Tbsp apple cider vinegar

- 2tsp sea salt

- 1Tsp ground black pepper

DIRECTIONS:

1. Preheat your air fryer to 200 degrees F.

2. Place the cucumber slices on a paper towel and layer another paper towel on top to absorb the moisture in the cucumbers.

3. Place the dried slices in a large bowl and toss with the vinegar, ground black pepper, and salt.

4. Place the cucumber slices on a tray lined with parchment and then bake in the air fryer for 3 hours. The cucumbers will begin to curl and brown slightly.

5. Turn off the air fryer and let the cucumber slices cool inside the fryer (this will help them dry a little more).

6. Enjoy right away or store in an airtight container.

NUTRITION: Calories 16, Total Fat 0g, Saturated Fat 0g, Total Carbs 4g, Net Carbs 3g, Protein 1g, Sugar 2g, Fiber 1g, Sodium 34mg, Potassium 0g

29.   Easy Buttered-Mushroom Cakes

Preparation Time: 18 Minutes • Servings: 8

INGREDIENTS

- Flour-1 ½ tbsps

- Bread crumbs-1 tbsps

- Milk-14-ounces

- Chopped mushrooms-4-ounce

- 1yellow onion; chopped.

- Ground Nutmeg-½ tsp

- Olive oil-2 tbsps

- Butter-1 tbsps

- Seasoning-Salt and black pepper to the taste

DIRECTIONS:

1. With medium-high temperature, Heat up the butter
   in a pan, put onion and mushrooms; stir well, cook
   for 3 minutes, add flour then stir well again and put

off the heat.

2. Put milk gradually, seasoned with salt, pepper, and nutmeg, stir carefully and set aside to cool down completely.

3. Mix oil with bread crumbs and whisk in a bowl.

4. A spoonful of the mushroom filling should be added to breadcrumbs mix, coat well, shape patties out of this mix.

5. Transfer them in your air fryer's basket and cook for 8 minutes at 400°F.

6. Share among plates and serve.

30.   Delicious Beet Wedges Dish

Preparation Time: 25 Minutes • Servings: 4

INGREDIENTS

- 4beets washed, peeled and cut into large wedges

- Lemon juice-1 tsp

- Seasoning-Salt and black to the taste

- Olive oil-1 tbsps

- garlic cloves; minced

DIRECTIONS

1. Combine and mix beets with oil, salt, pepper, garlic and lemon juice in a bowl; toss well,

2. Place mixture in your air fryer's basket and cook for 15minutes at a temperature of 400°F.

3. Share beets wedges on plates and serve.

31.   Chili Lime Broccoli Crunch

Preparation time: 5 minutes • Cooking time: 6 Hours •

Servings: 4

INGREDIENTS

- 4cups broccoli florets, chopped into bite sized

    pieces

- 1Tbsp olive oil

- 1tsp sea salt

- 1tsp lime zest

- 1Tbsp lime juice

- 1tsp chili powder

DIRECTIONS:

1. Preheat your air fryer to 135 degrees F.

2. Wash and drain the broccoli florets.

3. Place the broccoli in a large bowl and toss with

    the olive oil, lime juice, lime zest and sea salt.

4. Add the broccoli to the basket of your air fryer or spread them in a flat layer on the tray of your air fryer (either option will work!).

5. Cook in the air fryer for about 6 hours, tossing the broccoli every hour or so to cook evenly. Essentially, you will be dehydrating the broccoli.

6. Once the broccoli is fully dried, remove it from the air fryer, toss with the chili powder, and then let cool. It will keep crisping as it cools.

7. Enjoy fresh or store in an airtight container for up to a month.

NUTRITION: Calories 62, Total Fat 3g, Saturated Fat 0g, Total Carbs 3g, Net Carbs 1g, Protein 2g, Sugar 1g, Fiber 2g, Sodium 647mg, Potassium 0g

32.   Zucchini Chips

Preparation time: 15 minutes • Cooking time: 4 Hours

•Servings: 8

INGREDIENTS

- 4cups very thin zucchini slices

- 2Tbsp olive oil

- 2tsp sea salt

DIRECTIONS:

1. Preheat your air fryer to 135 degrees F.

2. Toss the thin zucchini slices with the oil and sea salt.

3. Place the zucchini on the air fryer tray or in the air fryer basket.

4. Cook for 4 hours, tossing the zucchini occasionally to allow it to dehydrate evenly.

5. Once crisp, remove the zucchini from the air

fryer and enjoy!

NUTRITION: Calories 40, Total Fat 4g, Saturated Fat 0g, Total Carbs 3g, Net Carbs 2g, Protein 1g, Sugar 2g, Fiber 1g, Sodium 570mg, Potassium 0g

33.　Crustless Pizza

Preparation Time: 10 minutes • Servings: 1

INGREDIENTS

- 2slices sugar-free bacon; cooked and crumbled

- 7slices pepperoni

- ½ cup shredded mozzarella cheese

- ¼ cup cooked ground sausage

- 2tbsp. low-carb, sugar-free pizza sauce, for dipping

- 1tbsp. grated Parmesan cheese

DIRECTIONS

1. Cover the bottom of a 6-inch cake pan with mozzarella. Place pepperoni, sausage and bacon on top of cheese and sprinkle with Parmesan

2. Place pan into the air fryer basket. Adjust the temperature to 400 Degrees F and set the timer for

5 minutes.

3. Remove when cheese is bubbling and golden. Serve

warm with pizza sauce for dipping.

NUTRITION: Calories: 466; Protein: 28.1g; Fiber: 0.5g;

Fat: 34.0g; Carbs: 5.2g

34.   Olives and Zucchini Cakes

Preparation Time: 17 minutes • Servings: 6

INGREDIENTS

- 3spring onions; chopped.

- ½ cup kalamata olives, pitted and minced

- 3zucchinis; grated

- ½ cup parsley; chopped.

- ½ cup almond flour

- 1egg

- Cooking spray

- Salt and black pepper to taste.

DIRECTIONS

1. Take a bowl and mix all the ingredients except the cooking spray, stir well and shape medium cakes out of this mixture

2. Place the cakes in your air fryer's basket, grease them

with cooking spray and cook at 380°F for 6 minutes

on each side. Serve as an appetizer.

NUTRITION: Calories: 165; Fat: 5g; Fiber: 2g; Carbs:

3g; Protein: 7g

35.   Tomato Bites

Preparation Time: 25 minutes • Servings: 6

INGREDIENTS

- 6tomatoes; halved

- 2oz. watercress

- 3oz. cheddar cheese; grated

- 1tbsp. olive oil

- 3tsp. sugar-free apricot jam

- 2tsp. oregano; dried

- A pinch of salt and black pepper

DIRECTIONS

1. Spread the jam on each tomato half, sprinkle oregano, salt and pepper and drizzle the oil all over them

2. Introduce them in the fryer's basket, sprinkle the cheese on top and cook at 360°F for 20

minutes

3. Arrange the tomatoes on a platter, top each half with some watercress and serve as an appetizer.

NUTRITION: Calories: 131; Fat: 7g; Fiber: 2g; Carbs: 4g; Protein: 7g

36.   Spinach Rolls

Preparation Time: 26 minutes Servings: 6

INGREDIENTS:

- 3cups mozzarella; shredded

- 6oz. spinach; chopped.

- 4oz. cream cheese, soft

- ½ cup almond flour

- 2eggs; whisked

- ¼ cup parmesan; grated

- 2tbsp. ghee; melted

- 4tbsp. coconut flour

- A pinch of salt and black pepper

DIRECTIONS

1. Take a bowl and mix the mozzarella with coconut and almond flour, eggs, salt and pepper, stir well until you obtain a dough and roll it well on a

parchment paper

2. Cut into triangles and leave them aside for now

3. Take a bowl and mix the spinach with parmesan, cream cheese, salt and pepper and stir really well.

4. Divide this into the center of each dough triangle, roll and seal the edges

5. Brush the rolls with the ghee, place them in your air fryer's basket and cook at 360°F for 20 minutes

6. Servings as an appetizer.

NUTRITION: Calories: 210; Fat: 8g; Fiber: 1g; Carbs: 3g; Protein: 8g

37.   Ranch Roasted Almonds

Preparation Time: 11 minutes • Servings: 2 cups

INGREDIENTS ½ (1-oz. ranch) dressing mix packet

2cups raw almonds. 2tbsp. unsalted butter; melted.

DIRECTIONS

1. Take a large bowl, toss almonds in butter to evenly coat. Sprinkle ranch mix over almonds and toss. Place almonds into the air fryer basketAdjust the temperature to 320 Degrees F and set the timer for 6 minutes. Shake the basket two- or three-times during cookingLet cool at least 20 minutes. Almonds will be soft but become crunchier during cooling. Store in an airtight container up to 3 days.

NUTRITION: Calories: 190; Protein: 6.0g; Fiber: 3.0g; Fat: 16.7g; Carbs: 7.0g

CHAPTER 9

DESSERT

38.   Cashew Dip

Preparation time: 5 minutes• Cooking time: 12 minutes •

Servings: 6

INGREDIENTS

- 1cup cashews, soaked in water for 4 hours and drained 1cup heavy cream

- 1tablespoon lemon zest, grated

- 1tablespoon lemon juice

- A pinch of salt and black pepper

- 1tablespoon chives, chopped

DIRECTIONS

1. In a blender, combine all the ingredients, pulse well

and transfer to a ramekin.

2. Put the ramekin in your air fryer's basket and cook at 350 degrees F for 12 minutes.

3. Serve as a party dip.

NUTRITION: Calories 144, Fat 2, Fiber 1, Carbs 3, Protein 4

39.   Smoked Salmon Salad

Preparation time: 5 minutes • Cooking time: 10 minutes •

Servings: 4

INGREDIENTS:

- 4ounces smoked salmon, skinless, boneless and cubed
- 1cup kalamata olives, pitted and halved
- 1cup corn
- 1cup baby spinach
- 2tablespoons lemon juice
- 1teaspoon avocado oil
- 1tablespoon chives, chopped
- A pinch of salt and black pepper

DIRECTIONS

1. In the air fryer's pan, mix the salmon with the olives and the other ingredients, put the pan in

the machine and cook at 350 degrees F for 10 minutes.

2. Divide into bowls and serve as an appetizer.

NUTRITION: Calories 100, Fat 2, Fiber 1, Carbs 2, Protein 2

40.   Salmon Meatballs

Preparation time: 5 minutes • Cooking time: 20 minutes •

Servings: 6

INGREDIENTS

- 1pound salmon fillets, boneless, skinless and ground
- 2eggs, whisked
- ¼ cup almond flour
- ½ teaspoon sweet paprika
- 1teaspoon garlic powder
- A pinch of salt and black pepper
- 1tablespoon parsley, chopped
- Cooking spray

DIRECTIONS

1. In a bowl, mix the salmon with the eggs and the other ingredients except the cooking spray,

stir well and shape medium meatballs out of this mix.

2. Pace them in your lined air fryer's basket, grease with cooking spray and cook at 360 degrees F for 20 minutes.

3. Serve as an appetizer.

NUTRITION: Calories 180, Fat 5, Fiber 2, Carbs 5, Protein 7

41.   Chicken Meatballs

Preparation time: 5 minutes • Cooking time: 20 minutes •

Servings: 8

INGREDIENTS

- 1and ½ pounds chicken breast, skinless, boneless and ground
- 2eggs, whisked
- 1tablespoon oregano, chopped
- 1tablespoon chives, chopped
- ¼ cup almond flour
- A pinch of salt and black pepper
- 2garlic cloves, minced
- 2spring onions, chopped
- Cooking spray

DIRECTIONS

1. In a bowl, mix the meat with the eggs and the

other ingredients except the cooking spray, stir well and shape medium meatballs out of this mix.

2. Arrange the meatballs in your air fryer's basket, grease them with cooking spray and cook at 360 degrees F for 20 minutes.

3. Serve as an appetizer.

NUTRITION: Calories 257, Fat 14, Fiber 1, Carbs 3, Protein 17

42.   Ginger Dip

Preparation time: 5 minutes • Cooking time: 20 minutes •

Servings: 6

INGREDIENTS

- 1cup Greek yogurt

- ½ cup heavy cream

- 2tablespoons ginger, grated

- 2shallots, chopped

- 1tablespoon chives, chopped

- A pinch of salt and black pepper

- Cooking spray

DIRECTIONS:

1. In the air fryer's pan, mix the cream with the yogurt and the other ingredients, put the pan in the machine and cook at 380 degrees F for 20 minutes.

2   Serve as a party dip.

NUTRITION: Calories 200, Fat 12, Fiber 2, Carbs 3,

Protein 14

43.   Asparagus and Olives Bowls

Preparation time: 5 minutes • Cooking time: 15 minutes •

Servings: 8

INGREDIENTS

- ½ pound asparagus, roughly chopped

- 1cup black olives, pitted and halved

- 1cup kalamata olives, pitted and halved

- 1cup baby spinach

- Juice of 1 lime

- 2tablespoons olive oil

- A pinch of salt and black pepper

DIRECTIONS

1. In the air fryer's pan, mix the asparagus with the olives and the other ingredients, put the pan in the machine and cook at 390 degrees F for 15 minutes.

2 Divide into bowls and serve as an appetizer.

NUTRITION: Calories 173, Fat 4, Fiber 2, Carbs 3, Protein 6

44. Walnuts and Radish Bites

Preparation time: 5 minutes • Cooking time: 15 minutes •

Servings: 4 INGREDIENTS

- 1pound radishes, halved

- 1cup walnuts

- 1teaspoon chili powder

- 1teaspoon sweet paprika

- A pinch of salt and black pepper

- 2tablespoons avocado oil

DIRECTIONS:

1. In the air fryer's basket, mix the radishes with the walnuts and the other ingredients, toss and cook at 400 degrees F for 15 minutes.

2. Serve as a snack.

NUTRITION: Calories 174, Fat 5, Fiber 1, Carbs 3,

Protein 6

45.   Bread pudding

Preparation Time: 1 hour 10 Minutes • Servings: 4

INGREDIENTS

- Glazed doughnuts: 6 crumbled

- Cherries: 1 cup

- Egg yolks: 4

- Sugar: ¼ tbsp

- Chocolate chips: ½ cup.

- Whipping cream: 1 ½ cups

- Raisins: ½ cup

DIRECTIONS

1. Mix cherries, egg yolks and whipping cream in a bowl A then stir well.

2. Mix raisins, sugar, chocolate chips and doughnuts in another bowl B and stir

3. Combine the contents of bowl A and bowl B

4. Place them in a greased pan and cook for 1 hour at 310 ° F let it cool then serve.

NUTRITION: Calories: 302; Fat: 8; Protein: 10; Carbohydrates: 23; Fiber: 2

46.　　Almond and Cocoa Cake

reparation time: 10 minutes • Cooking time: 30 minutes

• Servings: 8

INGREDIENTS:

- 1and ½ cup stevia

- 1cup flour

- ¼ cup cocoa powder+ 2 tablespoons

- ½ cup chocolate almond milk

- 2teaspoons baking powder

- 2tablespoons canola oil

- 1teaspoon vanilla extract

- 1and ½ cups hot water

- Cooking spray

DIRECTIONS

1. In a bowl, mix flour with 2 tablespoons

   cocoa, baking powder, almond milk, oil and

vanilla extract, whisk well and spread on the bottom of a cake pan greased with cooking spray.

2. In a separate bowl, mix stevia with the rest of the cocoa and the water, whisk well and spread over the batter in the pan.

3. Introduce in the fryer and cook at 350 degrees F for 30 minutes.

4. Leave the cake to cool down, slice and serve.

5. Enjoy!

NUTRITION: Calories 250, Fat 4, Fiber 3, Carbs 10, Protein 2

47.   Blueberry Cake

Preparation time: 10 minutes • Cooking time: 30 minutes •Servings: 6

INGREDIENTS

- ½ cup whole wheat flour
- ¼ teaspoon baking powder
- ¼ teaspoon stevia
- ¼ cup blueberries
- 1/3 cup almond milk
- 1teaspoon olive oil
- 1teaspoon flaxseed, ground
- ½ teaspoon lemon zest, grated
- ¼ teaspoon vanilla extract
- ¼ teaspoon lemon extract
- Cooking spray

DIRECTIONS

1. In a bowl, mix flour with baking powder, stevia, blueberries, milk, oil, flaxseeds, lemon zest, vanilla extract and lemon extract and whisk well.

2. Spray a cake pan with cooking spray, line it with parchment paper, pour cake batter, introduce in the fryer and cook at 350 degrees F for 30 minutes.

3. Leave the cake to cool down, slice and serve.

4. Enjoy!

NUTRITION: Calories 210, Fat 4, Fiber 4, Carbs 10, Protein 4

48.   Peach Cinnamon Cobbler

Preparation time: 10 minutes • Cooking time: 30 minutes • Servings: 4

INGREDIENTS

- 4cups peaches, peeled and sliced
- ¼ cup coconut sugar
- ½ teaspoon cinnamon powder
- 1and ½ cups vegan crackers, crushed
- ¼ cup stevia
- ¼ teaspoon nutmeg, ground
- ½ cup almond milk
- 1teaspoon vanilla extract
- Cooking spray

DIRECTIONS

1. In a bowl, mix peaches with coconut sugar and cinnamon and stir.

2. In a separate bowl, mix crackers with stevia, nutmeg, almond milk and vanilla extract and stir.

3. Spray a pie pan that fits your air fryer with cooking spray and spread peaches on the bottom.

4. Add crackers mix, spread, introduce into the fryer and cook at 350 degrees F for 30 minutes

5. Divide the cobbler between plates and serve.

6. Enjoy!

NUTRITION: Calories 201, Fat 4, Fiber 4, Carbs 7, Protein 3

49.   Easy Pears Dessert

Preparation time: 10 minutes • Cooking time: 25 minutes • Servings: 12 INGREDIENTS

- 6big pears, cored and chopped
- ½ cup raisins 1teaspoon ginger powder
- ¼ cup coconut sugar
- 1teaspoon lemon zest, grated

DIRECTIONS

1. In a pan that fits your air fryer, mix pears with raisins, ginger, sugar and lemon zest, stir, introduce in the fryer and cook at 350 degrees F for 25 minutes.

2. Divide into bowls and serve cold.

3. Enjoy!

NUTRITION: Calories 200, Fat 3, Fiber 4, Carbs 6, Protein 6

50. **Strawberry Cheesecake**

Preparation time: 10 minutes • Cooking time: 20 minutes • Servings: 4

INGREDIENTS

- 2cups cream cheese, soft
- 1cup strawberries, chopped
- ½ teaspoon almond extract
- 2eggs, whisked
- 4tablespoons sugar
- 1cup graham cookies, crushed
- 2tablespoons butter, melted

DIRECTIONS

1. In a bowl, mix the cookies with the butter and press this on the bottom of a lined cake pan.

2. In a bowl, mix the cream cheese with the rest of the ingredients, whisk, spread this over the crust and

cook your cheesecake in your air fryer at 310 degrees F for 20 minutes.

3. Cool the cheesecake down and keep in the fridge for a few hours before serving.

NUTRITION: Calories 195, Fat 12, Fiber 4, Carbs 20, Protein 7

51. Cherries and Rhubarb Bowls

Preparation time: 10 minutes • Cooking time: 25 minutes • Servings: 4

INGREDIENTS

- 2cups cherries, pitted and halved
- 1cup rhubarb, sliced
- 1cup apple juice
- 2tablespoons sugar
- ½ cup raisins.

DIRECTIONS

1. In a pan that fits your air fryer, combine the cherries with the rhubarb and the other ingredients, toss, cook at 330 degrees F for 35 minutes, divide into bowls, cool down and serve.

NUTRITION: Calories 212, Fat 8, Fiber 2, Carbs 13, Protein 7

52.   Chocolate Chips Cream

Preparation time: 10 minutes • Cooking time: 15 minutes • Servings: 4 INGREDIENTS

- 1cup coconut cream 2tablespoons sugar

- 1tablespoon cocoa powder

- 1teaspoon cinnamon powder

- 1cup heavy cream

- 1cup chocolate chips

DIRECTIONS:

1. In a bowl, mix the cream with the sugar and the other ingredients, whisk and divide into 4 ramekins.

2. Put the ramekins in the air fryer, cook at 340 degrees F for 15 minutes and serve cold.

NUTRITION: Calories 190, Fat 2, Fiber 1, Carbs 6, Protein 3

DAY MEAL PLAN

DAY	BREAKFAST	MAINS	DESSERTS
1.	Stuffed Portobello Mushrooms with Ground Beef	Indian Chickpeas	Butter Cookies
2.	Basil-Spinach Quiche	White Beans with Rosemary	Cream Cheese and Zucchinis Bars
3.	Stuffed Chicken Roll with Mushrooms	Squash Bowls	Coconut Cookies
4.	Eggs on Avocado Burgers	Cauliflower tew with Tomatoes and Green Chilies	Lemon Cookies
5.	Applesauce Mash with Sweet Potato	Simple Quinoa Stew	Delicious cheesecake
6.	Bacon and Kale Breakfast Salad	Green Beans with Carrot	Macaroons
7.	Fish Fritatta	Chickpeas and Lentils Mix	Amaretto and bread dough
8.	Spinach Frittata	Garlic Pork Chops	Orange cake
9.	Kale Quiche with Eggs	Honey Ginger Salmon	Apple bread

		Steaks	
10.	Olives Rice Mix	Mustard Pork Balls	Strawberry pie
11.	Sweet Quinoa Mix	Beef Meatballs in Tomato Sauce	Bread pudding
12.	Creamy Almond Rice	Green Stuffed Peppers	Pomegranate and chocolate bars
13.	Chives Quinoa Bowls	Sweet & Sour Chicken Skewer	Crisp apples
14.	Potato Casserole	Lamb Meatballs	Cocoa cookies
15.	Turkey and Peppers Bowls	Spiced Green Beans with Veggies	Strawberry shortcakes
16.	Turkey Tortillas	Chipotle Green Beans	Lentils and dates brownies
17.	Avocado Eggs Mix	Tomato and Cranberry Beans Pasta	Chocolate cookies
18.	Maple Apple Quinoa	Mexican Casserole	Mini lava cakes
19.	Chopped Kale with Ground Beef	Spicy Herb Chicken Wings	Banana bread
20.	Bacon Wrapped Chicken Fillet	Roasted Cauliflower with Nuts & Raisins	Granola
21.	Egg Whites with Sliced Tomatoes	Red Potatoes with Green	Tomato cake

		Beans and Chutney	
22.	Beef Balls with Sesame and Dill	Simple Italian Veggie Salad	Chocolate cake
23.	Zucchini Rounds with Ground Chicken	Spiced Brown Rice with Mung Beans	Coffee cheesecakes
24.	Meatball Breakfast Salad	Eggplant and Tomato Sauce	Fried banana
25.	Tomatoes with Chicken	Lemony Endive Mix	Banana cake
26.	Cherry Tomatoes Fritatta	Lentils and Spinach Casserole	Espresso cream and pears
27.	Whisked Eggs with Ground Chicken	Scallions and Endives with Rice	Lime cheesecakes Wrapped Pears
28.	Breakfast Bacon Hash	Cabbage and Tomatoes	Strawberry cobbler
29.	Eggplant and weet Potato Hash	Lemon Halibut	Almond and cocoa bars
30.	Eggs in Avocado	Medium-Rare Beef Steak	Ginger cheesecake
31.	Spaghetti Squash Casserole Cups	Fried Cod & Spring Onion	Plum cake

CPSIA information can be obtained
at www.ICGtesting.com
Printed in the USA
BVHW091141060521
606650BV00010B/1374